Weight Loss

Learn How To Lose 7 Lbs in 7 Days. Simple
Diet Plan To Start Losing Weight Right Now!

Table of content

Introduction

Your alarm is going off again. Another day filled with work, errands, family time, and chores. You live a life that you love, and it is true that you wouldn't change a thing about it, but then you look in the mirror.

Where did that weight come from? You ask yourself. It isn't as though it is anything drastic, but then you notice that your clothes aren't fitting like they used to. Time to hit the gym.

But who has time for that? You are already stretched thin trying to get the rest of your work done, and it is a top priority to be hanging out with your family, so how on earth are you now supposed to squeeze in gym time?

Something is being squeezed, all right, and it isn't your pants that have shrank. Don't worry, this book is your little super hero of dieting. Showing you easy to follow weight watchers tips that you can start now, we promise you that you will lose 7 pounds in 7 days, and you won't have to spend a single hour in the gym.

Using methods and tips that are proven to work, these things are all so easy you will wonder why you never did them before. Your energy will go up, and you will find that you are sleeping better at night as well.

Your waistline will thank you, and all you have to do is eat right and exercise a little bit. It isn't hard and we promise you it isn't going to hurt your body or your budget.

Fast, simple, inexpensive, and easy to follow, this diet plan is so easy you won't have a problem following it for as long as you need to, and what makes it even better is that the results are real. What are you waiting for? With something this easy right in front of you, you have absolutely nothing to lose.

Get ready for a new and transformed you, and you will be thrilled to show off your new bod in a week, and find it easier than ever to continue this diet until you are the size that you always wanted to be!

Chapter 1 – Why It Works

This is a program that promises results, and that is not something that is to be taken lightly. When you are devoting your time and health to something, it is important to know for sure that it is going to work, and this is no exception.

There are times when the facts don't matter so much as the reason behind the facts. If someone were to ask you why your weight loss plan works, and you didn't have an answer, they would probably plant speculation in your mind, because weight loss has become so scientific these days that people want to know and verify what they are doing before they do it.

This is not a bad idea, after all, if you are going to spend your money on something, you want to know that it works, and how are you going to know that if you don't know why?

The answer is simple. This is not a fad diet, and it is not crash dieting. It is a plan that will incorporate your actual lifestyle with a weight loss plane, and as a result, leave you with something that you can continue to follow throughout your life, and eliminate your stressing as well as your battle with your weight.

Once you know how this works, you will be able to take your dieting past the realm of this book, and be able to apply it to real life situations that you will face, and now that you will be able to face and make the right decisions.

There is no wrong way to diet, but there is an effective way, and an ineffective way, and we are here to show you what ways work. Don't worry, it isn't anything that is hard or painful, and you don't have to be that person that stands in the grocery store for hours trying to decide what you can and can't have.

That doesn't work, because you live a real life that is full of a variety of foods. You need a diet that is going to be understanding of your real lifestyle, and one that you are able to stick with no matter what is thrown your way.

When you reach the end of this book, not only will you be able to lose 7 pounds in a week, you won't have to worry what party you attend, what restaurant you eat at, or if there happens to be cupcakes at work.

This is an all-encompassing plant that will keep you losing weight, healthy, and a fitter, thinner version of you that you always wanted to be, without depriving yourself of a single frosted donut.

Chapter 2 – The Breakfast Battle

Breakfast is the most important meal of the day. That is a phrase that we are all familiar with, whether it was something that you saw on the TV, or if it was what your mother told you when you told her you didn't have time.

But that was true then, and it still is. Breakfast is the most important meal, and many of us skip it because we feel that we do not have time for it. The awful truth is that skipping breakfast may be one of the biggest road blocks you are facing when you are trying to lose weight.

This is because breakfast is what wakes up your metabolism. Yes, that sleeping metabolism doesn't like to wake up just like the rest of you, so you need to give it a jump start every morning, and coffee doesn't cut it.

You don't need a lot, although an actual meal for breakfast is really the most ideal thing that you can do. If you are insistent that you do not have time, and that you firmly believe that you don't, here are a few things that you can do that will give you a fast and easy breakfast in the morning, and jump start that metabolism for the whole day.

Eat a handful of almonds, and a banana.

Tossing back a handful of nuts and eating a banana doesn't take any time at all, and it really is enough to get that metabolism going. You can set out the nuts and banana on the counter the night before, and come morning all you have to do is reach over and grab it on your way out the door.

It's as simple as peeling a banana, and it is impossible that you don't have time to do that.

The never fail breakfast smoothie.

If you have a few more minutes than the old nut and banana method, and if you would like to enjoy breakfast a little bit more, try a smoothie. They are simple, easy to make, and easy to eat on the run.

Toss a smoothie in your cup and you are ready for the rest of the day, and all you had to do was throw a few ingredients in the blender on your way by. Here are a couple of low calorie, tasty smoothies that you can make in a few minutes, and not have to worry about time or effort.

Banana Smoothie:

4 ice cubes

1 tablespoon honey

1 banana

1 cup milk

Toss all of the ingredients in the blender, and turn on. When smooth, pour into your mug and you are ready to go! Something that is that easy to make and tastes too good is way too good to pass up.

Your waistline will be thanking you for the added boost that you are providing, and you will be more alert and better off at work if you eat in the morning anyway.

Scrambled Egg Mug

2 eggs

Splash of milk

Salt and pepper

Cheese is optional

Combine everything in a coffee mug and place in the microwave for 45 seconds. When finished, fluff with fork and add cheese if desired. Let stand for one minute, and there you have it, another easy breakfast that took less than 5 minutes to make.

I know it is tough to include breakfast into your morning routine, but trust me, it is going to be well worth your time. Our bodies are funny in that they need some calories in the morning to help them burn more calories in the afternoon, but as odd as it sounds, it really is effective.

Never skip another breakfast, and you will be happy to see the results showing within a couple of days.

Chapter 3 – Overcoming the Lunchtime Craze

It is a well-known fact that many of us skip breakfast, and as a result many of us then over eat at lunch time due to the fact you are starving. It does start to create a vicious cycle of skipping one meal to save on calories, then over indulging on the next meal.

The negative result is two-fold in that your metabolism isn't working as well as it should be due to not getting breakfast, and the fact that you have now eaten more calories than you wanted to so it has more to deal with.

This, of course, isn't your fault in that you have only been told that calories are the bad guys and you need to avoid those pesky little monsters to keep from getting fat. But the opposite is actually true.

It is time to reinvent the way you view calories, and the way your body uses them. Calories do not equal fat, and you do need them to get through your day. To get through your life, really, they are just that important.

Think of calories not as something that is producing fat, but as something that is giving you energy. Too much of this fuel is what results in you gaining weight, but in and of themselves they are as harmless as anything.

Calories in equals fuel into your body, and it is up to you to burn off that fuel and be ready for the next round of fuel that is going in. This is why we are looking for foods that are low calorie, but are high in nutrients for you to eat.

You will not be putting in more fuel than you are going to use, but at the same time you are going to be feeling full. Getting a lot of nutrition while skimping on the calories is like getting the most bang for your buck.

Now, there is the concept of good calories versus bad calories, and how you are to come to terms with each, but we will talk more about that later. Now we are going to look at the lunchtime craze, and what you can do to avoid undoing your morning when you get here.

Lunch should be simple, but high in protein as much as you can. This is both the pick me up from the morning as well as what needs to get you through to dinner. Health and high protein is the name of the game when it comes to lunch.

You don't want to mess up the day because you are weak from hunger, and a lot of the time it is when you give up on the rest of the day. With the all-too-common all or nothing attitude, a lot of people feel like they need to give up on the rest of the day as soon as they stumble.

So what should you be looking at for lunch? Something simple. Think salmon fillets, eggs, peanut butter... or any nut butter for that matter. Nuts are a staple, and don't be afraid of things like milk. It doesn't matter if it is dairy, nut, or coconut, milk is your friend.

Try this:

Salmon Filet on Rice with Broccoli

Salmon fillet

½ cup cooked white rice

1 tablespoon butter

½ cup broccoli

Grill the salmon filet (or have it done the night before, this will save time the next day if you are short on time.) Top the rice with the butter, and the salmon fillet, serve with the steamed broccoli alongside.

This is a more elaborate dish for lunch, but at the same time it remains simple, and that is a huge benefit to what we are showing you.

You can still have tasty and delicious things for lunch, while watching your weight. It is truly a win for you and your taste buds.

This is simple and delicious, and will only take minutes to put together, you will also have the great benefit of staying full through dinner time, and you won't have to feel guilty about the lunch.

This is not a diet of depravation, you won't get anywhere if you deprive yourself. What you need to do is find some things that you like, that you can then replace the unhealthy things in your diet with these healthy things.

It is not a bad thing to indulge yourself from time to time, but what you need to do is find a balance between what is healthy and what isn't. You can have whatever you want, whenever you want it, and that is just what this program is about.

Once you have been able to achieve this balance, you will find a level of freedom in your diet, and the weight will start to melt off. When you get to dinner in your day, you will find that it is really more of a victorious wrap up to how the rest of the day went.

Chapter 4 – How to Guiltlessly Indulge

Now we have to take a look at dinner. This is the final wrap up to the day (except for dessert, of course, but that is considered extra!) So let's look at a way that you can use this to your ultimate benefit.

There is a lot you can do when it comes to dinner, especially if you have had a good day with the rest of your diet. And if you haven't, don't sweat it, tomorrow is a new day, and there is no need to blow the rest of your day, either.

No matter what you did on the last meal, remember that each new meal is a new opportunity to do better than you did the previous meal. That is one of the benefits of this kind of diet.

You are free to eat whatever you want whenever you want, as long as you keep calories in mind. If you want to eat dessert, do it, but don't eat a lot of it. Dinner is another matter, of course, and that is what you want to enjoy most in your day.

We didn't include a recipe for dinner, because you have so many options that you can do, so let's take a look at the rules that you need to follow in order to keep in your caloric guide and still lose that weight that you want to lose.

Let's first back up a few steps, and take a look at what caloric intake is, and why it is important to follow. Like we were talking about before, calories are energy, and it is the extra calories that the body takes in that it later turns to fat if it is not used.

So what is the right amount of calories for you to intake? Well, this has some determining factors that only you can decide. First of all, are you active? What is your starting weight? What kind of job do you work?

Why are of these important? Because all of these things factor in to how many calories you are burning throughout the day, and how many you can have for the rest of your day.

There are countless online calculators that all factor in how many calories you are burning based on a certain activity you engage in during your day, and how many calories you can consume based on what you are doing.

You will really be surprised at how many calories you are allowed in a day, and how much you can consume for that amount of calories.

If you are careful to watch your intake, and know what you are consuming, you will be able to eat what you like and whenever you like it.

This is going to be such a relief to your whole diet, and the whole way you get to live your life. Learn the daily intake amounts that the FDA recommends, and follow those, and your weight will basically melt off of you.

To make this even simpler for you, we have included some simple and rule of thumb methods that you can follow that will help you get rid of the weight while not compromising what is good for you, and for your weight loss.

There are 3500 calories in 1 pound of fat. And that is the amount that you need to burn to lose weight.

Yes, this may sound like a lot at first, especially when you are thinking in terms of burning this amount in a single week, but don't worry, we are going to look into exercising and how that will relate to your weight loss in the next chapter.

For now, let's look at what it means for portion control.

If you don't want to take the time to sit at the grocery store and figure out how many calories are in a single serving, then you need to learn what the common portion size is for a meal, and how that relates to what the packaging tells us when they are talking about serving sizes.

Insider's Tip: A serving size and a portion size are two different things. A serving size is the premeasured amount that the company has measured and calculated the corresponding caloric count

A portion size is the amount that you should be eating for your meal. As a rule of thumb, this is roughly half a cup of cooked grains or vegetables, a s 6 or 8 ounce portion of meat, and fruit that is roughly equivalent to your fist size.

If you are curious as to how many calories are in any of these things, you should look them up online. There are so many variables to what you are having that it would be difficult to give you an actual caloric amount that would be accurate.

Make sure, however, that you are always eating until you are full, but that you stop as soon as you feel full. Never eat to the point that you feel stuffed, and always leave a small amount on your plate. This is a visible reminder that you are in control of what you are eating, and that you eat to live, and don't live to eat.

Once you have this all under control, you don't have to worry about what you are eating so much anymore. This is because you are only eating a reasonable portion, and since you are eating healthy foods most of the time, you are balancing out the bad food that is trying to creep in.

Chapter 5 – Shake it Off

Ultimately, in spite of everything that you have been told, it is diet rather than exercise that determines your weight issue. Sure, if you want to have all of those defined abs, or that toned physique, you are going to have to exercise, but it is what you eat, and how much of it that you eat that determines what you weigh.

For example, back in the nineties when it was the trend to be as skinny as one could be, there was little exercise going on, it was women that didn't eat much. Mind you this is a terrible and unhealthy way to be, and we never recommend that you starve yourself, but the point is weight loss comes from food rather than exercise.

Exercise serves many wonderful and beneficial purposes to you, and for health you should strive to engage in some form of aerobic activity for at least 20 minutes a day, 3 days a week.

What is interesting about this standard, however, is that the health that they are referring to actually is for muscle, bone, heart, and joint just as much as it is for weight loss.

What you must also realize is that you don't have to do those exercises that require you to do backbreaking work. A brisk walk in the park, or a simple jog around your neighborhood will do the trick.

Moderate exercise with a lot of water is proven to help you lose more weight than the intense exercises, and it is something that you will be able to enjoy doing, so there won't be any worries that exercising will feel like a chore after the first week of doing it.

If you will notice, on the sides of any exercise equipment, it says that diet and exercise are what play a factor in what you weigh and how you feel.

Exercise is what shapes you into a certain thing, diet is what determines how fast that goes as well as what you ultimately weigh.

This is also why there are people out there that exercise regularly and are still on the overweight side of the scale.

This goes to what we were just talking about. Sure, they will have healthier hearts and muscles and such than those that do not exercise, but they will also weigh more because of what they are eating.

If that is what works for them, and if that is what makes them happy, then they should do it, but what does that have to do with what we are talking about?

For starters, you need to start an exercise regime. And for that regime we are shooting for health, so we recommend that you do what is recommended for health. 20 minutes a day 3 days a week. Don't do all of these days in a row, every other day during the week is fine.

Now, for the weight loss that we promised, you need to look at what you are eating. Take a day and measure the foods that you consume, and calculate the amount of calories you are taking in.

Once you have that figured out, figure out how many calories you burn in a work day, without including the exercise. Now that you have all of these figures, you can do the math to see how many calories you need to burn to lose the weight that you want to lose.

Don't be discouraged if the number is high. For starters, we are now looking at healthier eating, along with portion control. What this means is that there is going to be a lot fewer calories going into your body.

Added to that is the fact that you are now exercising. That means there is that boost of caloric burn 3 times a week that you were not getting before. Meaning that there is that much more calories getting burned and more weight coming off.

You are going to be amazed at how quickly the weight melts off of you at first. It will feel great to see the number coming down on the scale, and in a matter of days you will feel a lot better, have more energy, and be able to sleep better.

It is almost magical how much better you feel with even a couple of pounds burned off, but that is just the beginning. Once you get the ball rolling, and embrace your new lifestyle, there will be no stopping you.

You will find that it only gets easier to say no to the food that was causing you problems, and to be able to control your portion sizes better. You will find that exercise even becomes so common place that you will wonder that you waited this long to do it.

Those pesky pounds will just drift away, and you will be into those jeans you have been saving in no time at all... maybe even by the end of this week!

Follow our guidelines daily, don't skip on breakfast, and make sure you get your exercise in at least a few times a week, and we promise you will see the results that you want to see in a matter of days, and that those results are going to last.

Look out world, this leopard has found her spots, and she knows that she can do anything. Now get out there and show them what you're made of, and that you can do anything you set your mind to doing.

Chapter 6 – Watching Your Weight for Life

Now that you have the answers, you are armed and dangerous. You know what to expect, and how to combat whatever comes your way. Friends and family are all going to be amazed at what you are able to accomplish in such a short amount of time, and they are going to be impressed when you are able to keep it off.

You won't have to be that person that doesn't eat at a party, yet you will still be that person that is losing the weight that they want to lose, and not stressing about how they are going to do it.

When you are able to apply these methods and these rules to your real life, you will be thrilled at the results. Remember to drink your smoothies at least every couple of days, and that you don't have to say no to sweets all of the time.

It's nice that you will see results so suddenly, as it is the first week that is the hardest. Once you are used to this kind of eating and lifestyle, it will become a second nature to you and you will just do it out of habit... and preference.

Food that you once thought you couldn't get enough of will begin to seem too sweet or have too much grease, and you won't have to do a thing to change that. This is because your body was designed to eat healthy foods, and it will want to do that whenever it is available.

I know that sounds crazy at first, but trust us, when you get to the point that you only have something sweet every now and then, you will know what we are talking about.

Exercise can be fun if you are doing what is right for you, and there are countless ways you can make the food that you love healthier and better for you. And remember, it is never a bad thing to treat yourself every now and then. No matter what you are thinking about it right now, you can do it, and you will see the results that you want.

It isn't hard and it isn't expensive, and it is really worth your time and efforts. Stick with this diet plan, even when you feel like giving up, and you will be happy that you didn't let a bad day stand in the way of a new and fit you.

Conclusion

There you have it, a diet plan that you can actually stick with, and one that is really effective. No more sweating it out in the gym, and no more browsing the internet for some diet plan that doesn't work and costs you a lot of money in the meantime.

So easy that you can follow it long after your first week, there is nothing stopping you from reaching your goal weight in a matter of weeks, and you will feel better both physically and emotionally.

Your confidence is going to soar as you are able to fit into those jeans that have been sitting in the back of your closet, and you will be happy to know that you are turning heads everywhere you go.

Nothing can hold you back, so get out there and face the world head on. You have what it takes to be great and live life to the fullest, so get out there and show them what you are made of.